MW00567062

Peace & Blessings.
Mike Ferserht

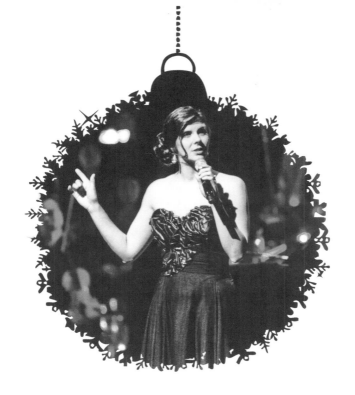

Ornament

• THE FAITH, JOY AND HOPE OF KRISTEN FERSOVITCH •

COMPILATION AND REFLECTIONS BY
ROBERT W. JONES

ORNAMENT
Written by Robert W. Jones
Copyright © 2015 by North Pointe Community Church

First edition. 1.00.
www.northpointechurch.ca

Printed in Canada

ISBN: 978-1-4866-0995-6

Word Alive Press
131 Cordite Road, Winnipeg, MB R3W 1S1
www.wordalivepress.ca

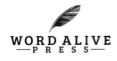 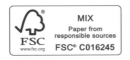

Cataloguing in Publication may be obtained through Library and Archives Canada

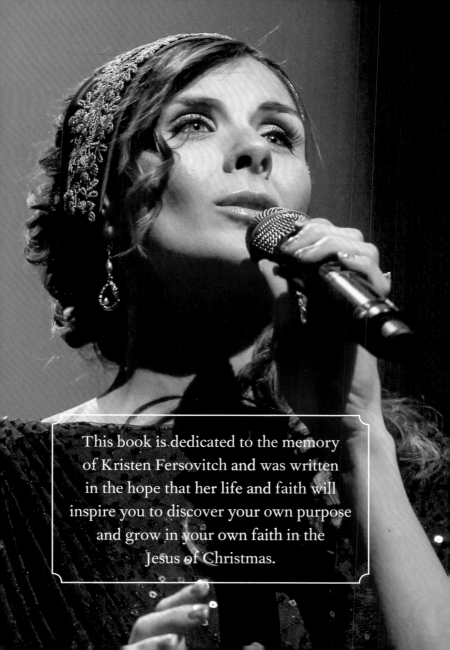

This book is dedicated to the memory of Kristen Fersovitch and was written in the hope that her life and faith will inspire you to discover your own purpose and grow in your own faith in the Jesus of Christmas.

She impacted the lives of many.

"In the face of unexpected and considerable adversity, Kristen was a model of faith and courage. It was impossible to spend time with her and not leave with a renewed awareness of the purpose and the people in your own life. Kristen was daily living out the words, "Rejoice always, pray continually, give thanks in all circumstances; for this is God's will for you in Christ Jesus."

(1 Thessalonians 5:16-18)

THE HONOURABLE MIKE LAKE, MP FOR EDMONTON MILLWOODS-BEAUMONT, HOUSE OF COMMONS, SEPTEMBER 27, 2011

"There was a peace she had that's hard to even understand. That has entirely to do with her faith and just trusting in God. She definitely found hope in her faith."

KENNEDY MILLER, KRISTEN'S SISTER

"In honor of a very dear friend who fought a courageous battle with cancer, Kristen, from this day forward I vow to do whatever I can to support your boys in any way I can. This is something I can do to honor and carry on your legacy. I love you! You will never be forgotten!"

CINDY KEATING, RED CARPET LIFE

"I called her my little sister. Kristen was so lovable, powerful, stubborn and opinionated—all the characteristics required to be a great performer. When I would spend time writing music with her and John, it was obvious when she didn't like something. Kristen wanted the audience to believe the message, not just be entertained by the music."

EMMANUEL FONTE, SINGING CHRISTMAS TREE CHOIR DIRECTOR

"She was beautiful and real and funny. She challenged us to live the best life we can, in the face of tragedy, in the face of despair. Not by telling us to, but by leading by example."

CARRIE DOLL, CTV NEWS, EDMONTON

"Kristen Fersovitch endured more hard times in the past four years than many people see in a lifetime, yet she remained unflappably happy."

ELIZABETH WITHEY, EDMONTON JOURNAL, DECEMBER 2011

"Here was a woman who was given a death sentence but chose to live life to its fullest and impact people in a positive way, daily. Women in recovery make a similar life decision to choose hope over the hopelessness they were in."

LERENA GREIG, EXTERNAL RELATIONS, EDMONTON DREAM CENTRE

"Thank you for arranging for Kristen and her sister and mother to sing. It was beyond words!!! I don't think anyone in the room had ever heard the Lord's Prayer sung so beautifully before."

ANN WIENS, THE *WHY* BOOK

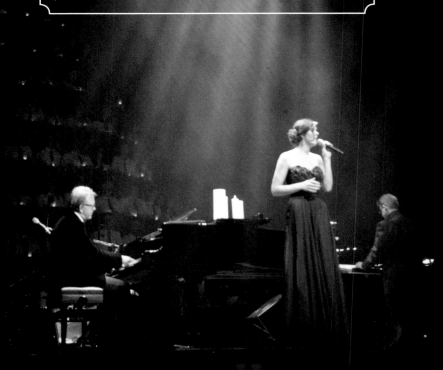

"Through this song and my journey I've gotten the opportunity to share my story of faith, joy and hope, even in the midst of life's hardships. God has taught me more than I could have ever imagined or dreamed through all of this."

KRISTEN FERSOVITCH

Emerging from her dressing room, she makes her way backstage. She fusses a bit with her dress to make sure it's properly situated, along with a shawl that's draped across her shoulder. She asks her sister how her hair looks and checks the mirror to see for herself. She's quite particular about the position of the scarf she has worked into her stylish hair.

I later come to realize that all the attention to shawls and scarves is simply an attempt to conceal the burn marks on her skin from the radiation therapy she's been receiving during the days leading up to tonight. She's right in the midst of the fight of her life—and yet she's here and ready to give her everything!

She walks out on the stage. She looks stunning and has a smile that lights up the room. Although she's fatigued from the treatments, she opens her heart and the room is instantly captivated. Her blue eyes tell a story before she ever sings a word. From the very beginning of a song she's penned, her spirit is poured out through every note and nuance, every lyric and look. I can tell she believes what she's singing, even though it has come at a cost. Her journey with cancer has been full of twists and turns, ups and downs, yet you know she's confident in who she is and who she belongs to.

After the show, I have the privilege of witnessing something even more amazing. I get to see this young woman completely engaged with her husband and little boys, loving and being loved immeasurably—so much so that it's contagious. It's no surprise to learn that she comes from a wonderful family of musicians who have spent their lives sharing the love of Jesus. Jesus is the lover of her soul, and without reservation she holds true to that love about which she has sung for years. In just a few short hours, this remarkable young woman makes an indelible impression upon me.

This describes my first encounter with Kristen Miller Fersovitch, and I, like so many others she impacted, am forever grateful.

Time is too slow, for those who wait
Time is too swift, for those who fear
Time is too long, for those who grieve
But for those who love and those who are loved
Time is eternity

Let this story of love, loss and unwavering faith in Christ remind you of the blessing of life and the absolute responsibility we have to make each second count for eternity.

This is your legacy living on, Kristen.

Mark Masri

Have you ever met someone and thought: there is a reason I am meeting this person? It's as if you had something to learn from them, they had something to teach you, but you had no idea what it was.

This is how I felt when I met Kristen. She was beautiful and real, funny and goofy, graceful and incredibly talented.

But it was her presence and her spirit that were larger than life. I wanted to be around her, to soak up her essence, to learn from her.

It was in December 2011 when I first heard the name Kristen Fersovitch. My dear friend John Cameron told me he was writing a song with one of the most amazing people he had ever met. He said her name was Kristen, she had three children, she was going to sing in The Tree, and she was battling terminal cancer. He told me she had changed his life and would impact countless others.

I was intrigued. I wanted to know who this person was that John had spoken so highly of.

A week before the 2011 edition of the Edmonton Singing Christmas Tree opened, CTV News decided to do a story about The Tree, and the young lady more and more people were talking about. Amanda Anderson from CTV News was our reporter. She's a hard-nosed journalist who has covered it all. But apparently not quite all, because when she came back to the newsroom that afternoon after interviewing Kristen, her eyes were red and swollen, and she stopped by my desk and simply said, "I've never met anyone like her. Come with me—you need to see this."

She played the interview and the video of John and Kristen singing, and the newsroom fell silent. There was something powerful in Kristen's presence and in her voice. And that was only the beginning. Because when Kristen took center stage at The Singing Christmas Tree to share her story, no one was quite prepared for what she was about to share, and the emotions she was about to evoke in everyone who heard her story. Her message was raw, truthful, and painful to listen to. She melted our hearts when she shared pictures of her husband Mike and her three beautiful boys, and she broke our hearts when she told us how sick she really was. And just when you felt you could bear no more, she started to sing. Her voice was pure and powerful, and she used phrases like "There's joy inside of you, something you cannot hide. It brings you hope, it brings you peace. It will come and change your life. 'Though your heart may be broken and your world may seem destroyed, it's Christmas time and you can find joy.'"

What? Joy when cancer is tearing you apart? Joy when the doctors tell you it's terminal? Joy when you look into the faces of your three young children, and know you may not be around to see them go to school, see them grow up, see them fall in love?

I stood backstage and I was frozen, and like every other person in that audience, I cried. I cried for Kristen, for her husband and boys, and their future. For her mom and dad and for her sister, for the future this tightknit family had to face.

And I cried because of all the things she forced me to think about. What is living really all about? How do you live a life of joy when your world is falling apart?

But she didn't see it that way. She stood on the stage and she sang her heart out, and as she did, she inspired everyone around her with her remarkable courage. She challenged us to live the best life we can in the face of tragedy, in the face of despair. Not by telling us to but leading by example. She was joy. And if she can choose it, in light of every challenge she was facing, the message is that all of us can.

This message resonated with everyone who saw her, and everyone who heard about her story. Her kindness and positivity was palpable. You could feel it. She made you feel grateful for everything you had in your life and you were motivated to be a better person.

After The Singing Christmas Tree wrapped up for the year, the emails started to pour in. I received countless messages and phone calls and was stopped on the street by people wanting to know "how Kristen was." People had connected with her and she had made an impact. They would follow up those questions with this comment, "It was the most powerful performance I have ever seen. I will never forget her. I have never cried so hard, and have been inspired so much all at the same time."

And so I brought her on CTV News to talk about the experience. She was so taken aback when I called her and asked for the interview. "Why?" she asked, her humility shining through. "Why would people want to hear from me? I'm just a big goof." And there lay the beauty of Kristen Fersovitch, and the power of her spirit: she moved us, she challenged us—without ever saying the words, without offering a piece of advice. She just lived it.

And she lived it for the next year, against all odds. Whenever you asked her where she got her strength from the, the answer was very clear. Her faith. It carried her through the darkest times and the most insurmountable challenges and brought her back to The Singing Christmas Tree stage in 2012. And she sang once more even as her health had really taken a turn for the worse.

When she showed up for The Tree, she was clearly in pain, although you'd never hear that from her. She had just finished an intense round of chemotherapy and radiation. She had lost a lot of her hair, so she wore a wig and made a headband the most fashionable accessory that year. Her chest was burned from radiation and the tumor in that area was painfully obvious. She knew it but wasn't phased by it— instead she talked about it with a sense of humor.

She came into my dressing room one night before the show wearing a cute little v-neck tee-shirt and said, "Look at this thing— AUGH, crazy thing, it's so itchy. Oh well, nothing a little high-necked dress won't fix." Then we'd sit 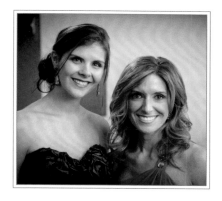 and talk like girlfriends. She'd try on my shoes, look at my clothes. We'd talk fashion, music and kids and life. When I asked what it was like to share the stage with Ruben Studdard, she said, "The guy can sing, he just can't remember the words!" When I asked her if she was going to wear her awesome Christian Louboutin shoes that year, she said her feet couldn't take it, kicked off her shoes and went barefoot on stage. At the end of the night when we were all exhausted, she still found the strength to go to the after show receptions, take pictures, meet people and spread the love. And she sang five sold-out shows, because people wanted to see Kristen Fersovitch.

How fitting it was that the theme of the show that year was "The Perfect Gift" because that's what Kristen gave all of us by coming back to that stage and singing one last time.

And as the song goes she wasn't scared to face her fears, she wasn't scared to spread her wings, she didn't mind that we shared her tears, because she taught us love is everything.

We saw it on stage and we felt it as she gave us and people she didn't know the perfect gift.

On one of the last nights that Kristen performed, I was standing backstage with her mom and dad. I looked over at them and tears were streaming down her dad's face. I said to him, "You must be so proud." He said, "You know, Carrie, just grateful, grateful for all the time we had with her."

Dave and Kathy, Kennedy, Mike, Lincoln, Tayven and Becket, thank you for sharing your daughter, your sister, your wife and your mommy with all of us. We too are grateful for everything Kristen taught us and for all the memories we have of her. I now know why I—and the rest of our community—was supposed to meet her and get to know Kristen Fersovitch. I think you all know it as well.

Today, as she smiles down on us, her legacy lives on.

If your heart hurts as you say goodbye, remember this. "If a small part of you is living the way she did, be grateful. Her spirit and her joy live on in you."

Carrie Doll

"I've got this joy in my heart,
something I cannot hide,
It brings me hope, it brings me peace
It's come and changed my life.
And though my heart may be broken
And my world may seem destroyed,
This precious child, He can bring joy."

With those words, Kristen Fersovitch sang her way into the hearts of thousands who attended the 2011 Singing Christmas Tree in Edmonton, Alberta, Canada. Facing inoperable cancer and a prognosis of mere months to live, she put her life on display for all to see. Kristen was a virtually unknown Canadian singer who shone as brightly as an American Idol on the biggest stage of her life. She became the most radiant light in The Singing Christmas Tree and in the hearts of countless people.

She said, "Through this song and my journey I've gotten the opportunity to share my story of faith, joy and hope, even in the midst of life's hardships. God has taught me more than I could have ever imagined or dreamed through all of this."

Music was Kristen's life. She was born into a musical family. When her mother Kathy Miller was pregnant with Kristen, she sang a duet with her husband Dave on Cross-

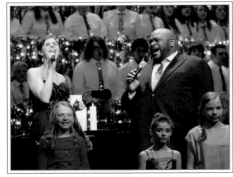

KRISTEN AND RUBEN STUDDARD

road's "100 Huntley Street" television program. The Millers travelled across North America singing gospel music in the early 80s. When Kristen was only two, they settled into Dave's hometown, Edmonton, Alberta. As she grew up, Kristen sang in choirs, trios, duets and worship teams, but she especially loved singing with her parents and sister, Kennedy. No family gathering was complete without a song. Thanksgiving celebrations concluded with an *a cappella* version of "Praise God from whom all blessings flow" and everybody had to participate. Kristen wanted everyone to sing with "all their might and heart."

Kristen was involved with the annual Singing Christmas Tree event in Edmonton all of her life, first as a child in the King's Kids choir, then as one of 150 adult singers, and eventually as a featured

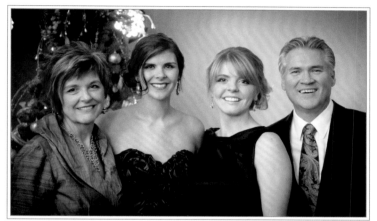

KATHY, KRISTEN, KENNEDY AND DAVE MILLER

soloist singing a song she co-wrote with The Singing Christmas Tree's executive producer and friend, John Cameron.

I first met Kristen when she was a seven-year-old in the Children's Ministry at Central Pentecostal Tabernacle (now North Pointe Community Church) where I have been a pastor since 1990. She grew up with our sons and was in our home as a teen as a part of youth group socials. I've stood with her backstage just before she sang in what we affectionately refer to as The Tree, when the performance was held at our church and again in her more recent performances at Edmonton's Jubilee Auditorium. Kristen welcomed me into her home and her hospital rooms. She invited me into her confidence and her heart. I felt like family hearing her say, "I love you."

Kristen participated in church, Sunday School, and youth group, and then as a young adult she volunteered for Youth With a Mission in Australia. She loved her parents, even if they butted heads at times. Kristen was popular with her peers. She had devoted, life-long friends. She was sincere, opinionated, passionate, headstrong, fun, talented, stubborn, edgy and endearing.

She married Mike Fersovitch, a firefighter. Together, they built their first two homes. Their firstborn son, Beckett, is disabled. They thought that might be the hardest experience they would face in life. Kristen gave birth to a second son but while pregnant with her third son she was diagnosed with inoperable cancer. The prognosis: less than two years to live. She was only 27.

She was a genuine believer in Jesus, but that didn't protect her from having doubts or questioning her faith. She wondered if God really loved her. Had she done something to deserve dying of cancer? How could she bear the thought of never seeing her boys grow up? But, even to her last breath, her refrain was, "I trust you Lord."

> Kristen loved the Christmas season and most of all the tradition of decorating her Christmas tree with ornaments.

When she was a little girl she dressed up in tree ornaments and asked her dad to take her picture. When she was a grown woman dressed up to sing in The Tree she was like a beautiful ornament, on display for all to see. In a tribute to Kristen's life, a star has been placed in The Singing Christmas Tree and shines through every performance as testimony to her inspirational courage.

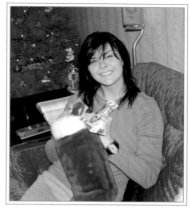

Ornament is a response to the many people who have asked, "How could I have a faith like Kristen's?" Each chapter features an ornament from the Fersovitch family Christmas tree and a related insight into Kristen's relationship with God. Kristen's own words are included too—both excerpts from her blog and conversations I had with her. At the end of each chapter are questions for you to reflect on what you have read and to help you grow in your own faith. I'm certain Kristen's desire would be for you to dig deeper into your own relationship with God.

"I tell you, whoever hears my word and believes him who sent me has eternal life and… has crossed over from death to life" (John 5:24).

Robert W. Jones

May 2015

CHAPTER 1

O, Christmas Tree

"Because that baby in a manger,
He made a path,
He made a way,
He'll bring you hope for tomorrow
And strength to face each day."

*"I bring you good news that will cause great joy for
all the people. Today in the town of David a Savior
has been born to you; he is the Messiah, the Lord."*

LUKE 2:10,11

Most Canadian children grow up with a Christmas tree in their house. Kristen grew up with a Christmas tree in her church! Central Tabernacle was home to The Singing Christmas Tree, an Alberta musical tradition. The pyramid-shaped roof of the church's sanctuary was designed to perfectly frame the six-story-high Tree. During Christmas season at Central Tabernacle, more than 13,000 people, some from around the world, would come to experience The Singing Christmas Tree. Often people had to be turned away at the doors because the seating capacity had been exceeded. Crowds started lining up ninety minutes before each presentation, sometimes standing in below zero, snowy weather.

When Kristen was five years old she made her vocal debut with the King's Kids Choir in The Singing Christmas Tree, singing and smiling in the front row of the choir. Behind her, nestled into the branches of the tree, were her mother, aunts, grandmother and friends of her family in the adult choir. The women dressed in white blouses with big red Christmas bows around their necks while the guys wore paisley vests with matching bow ties.

In Kristen's first year in The Singing Christmas Tree, the King's Kids Choir sang with a man and woman who performed a duet. During the dress rehearsal, Kristen took a liking to the man. As the kids practiced their entrance and exit cues, rehearsed their music and backed up the duet, Kristen watched the blond male singer and thought she'd like to sing with him one day.

On opening night the moment came for the King's Kids Choir to sing. The choir shuffled into their places, and the man and woman came on to sing their song. The house lights went up and the children saw hundreds of faces staring at them. Many of the other children struggled against their stage fright, but Kristen was in her element. She loved to perform. To the choir director, it seemed like the other kids had taken a step back as the duet began, but Kristen actually took a step forward. She was so enamoured with the male singer that she stepped out from her place with the choir and surprised him by taking hold of his hand. She made it a trio. The audience thought it was adorable.

> "This performance is His, for His Glory, for His name… because He is the one that has brought me the joy that I get to sing about."

Little did Kristen know that twenty-three Christmases later, in 2011, she would be standing on another stage in front of a sold-out auditorium, singing with the same man. The venue was now the Northern Alberta Jubilee Auditorium and the man was now the executive producer of the Edmonton Singing Christmas Tree, John Cameron.

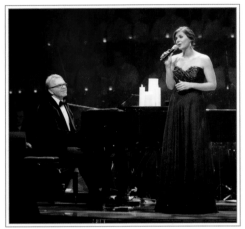

JOHN CAMERON AND KRISTEN, 2011 SINGING CHRISTMAS TREE

"The Tree," as it was often called, had been recognized by *Reader's Digest* as "*The* Christmas event in Canada." Kristen and John had co-written a song, which would help Kristen tell the story of what Christmas meant to her.

Kristen talked about how she felt on the day of the first performance. "Well, today's the big day. How am I feeling? Nervous? Yeah. Out my league? Maybe a little. But yet, when I think about it... I *grew up* singing in this thing. I was a little kid in the choir, and now there are still familiar faces from years ago everywhere I look, people who knew me as a little girl.

"One of my favourite things is that when I'm freaking out right before I hit the stage, it's my Uncle Bill who hands me my microphone. There's nothing like having family standing *right* with you before a big moment.

"Not much has changed about The Tree in terms of what's familiar to me except for location and really the audience is still the same: God. I get nervous about speaking and singing in front of thousands of people, but what's more nerve-racking: a group of people or singing for the one who created everything? This performance is His, for His Glory, for His name because *He* is the one that has brought me the joy that I get to sing about."

Kristen clearly understood that life was God's gift to her. Her gift to God was what she was making of her life. As much as it was in her power, she would make it a masterpiece.

Because that baby in a manger,
He made a path,
He made a way.
He'll bring you hope for tomorrow
And strength to face each day.
There is a Joy in my heart
Something I cannot hide
It brings me hope
It brings me peace
It's come and changed my life.

And though my heart may be broken,

And my world may seem destroyed,

That precious child,

He can bring JOY.

(Kristen Fersovitch/John Cameron)

REFLECTION

- Do you have a personal faith in Jesus as your Savior and God? Do you believe that Jesus loves you and died for you and was raised from the dead for you? Make a choice today to cross the "faith line." On one side of the line are people who know in their heads that Jesus exists, that He loves them and that he died for them. But to cross the faith line is to make those beliefs personal to you.

- What are your Christmas traditions? How does your faith play a part in those traditions?

Lord, I ask you to come into my life. I believe that you died for me and that you were raised to life from the dead. I ask you to forgive my sin and change me from the inside out. Give me a brand new start. I want to live the rest of my life for you, with your help. Thank you.

CHAPTER 2

Tinsel

"God IS love. It's who He is; it's what He does."

"*Whoever does not love does not know God, for God is love.*" 1 JOHN 4:8

Mike Fersovitch first saw Kristen when his cousin invited him to a Sunday evening service at Central Tabernacle. Kristen was on the platform, singing and Mike sat in the pew, smitten. He asked who the girl was. His cousin responded in no uncertain terms, "Forget that. You haven't got a chance. That's Kristen Miller."

A few years later, Mike and Kristen were dating, and he was again sitting in the pews while she was participating in The Singing Christmas Tree.

As it was every year, The Tree was adorned from top to bottom with tinsel – lots of shiny tinsel. Tinsel is a Tree tradition. On dress rehearsal night each choir member hangs strands of tinsel on the branches of The Tree near them. The producer is always very particular about how the tinsel is placed on The Tree because it's there for special effect.

On opening night at Central Tabernacle, the church would fill an hour early with people waiting in anticipation. Then the house lights would dim, the orchestra would start the overture and the choir would file into their rows. Just as the orchestra reached its crescendo, the choir would sing their first notes, the lights would come on full and the tinsel would catch the light, reflecting back a brilliance that caused the audience to gasp and then erupt in applause.

There were times during each performance when the choir had a break from singing. As they waited to sing again, some of the choir members would absentmindedly pick away at the tinsel, much to the chagrin of the choir director. But Kristen outdid them all.

The evening when Mike sat in the audience, Kristen pulled off the tinsel in her area, strand by strand and rolled the strands around in her hand. By the end of the night, the tree branches in her area were bare and she had created a little ball of hand-packed tinsel. She gave it to Mike after the performance as a memento of the evening. He still has it.

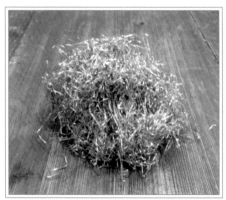

MIKE'S BALL OF TINSEL

At times, Kristen didn't feel God's love. She believed in God but she just didn't feel His closeness or approval. She often prayed to feel His love and there was nothing in response. Then, when her dis-appointment was at its peak, the light would come on. Just like the tinsel, God's love shone on everything. His love caught the light of Bible verses that Kristen read, and reflected joy back on her. It was brilliant.

> "I knew that God loved me. I *knew* it in my head. I have it highlighted, underlined and circled in my Bible."

"I knew that God loved me," Kristen said. "I *knew* it in my head. I have it highlighted, underlined and circled in my Bible.

"But the problem was, I never made it personal. Out of the hundreds of times I have sung 'Jesus loves me'… I realized that each time I was just singing words… I never actually thought of it as being *for me*.

"God loves *me*.

"And so… I am excited. I am entering into a new chapter of getting to know who God *really* is. A season of renewing my mind.

"When you open the Bible, love is all you see. Over and over again: God's love for people. My problem was I've been wanting God's love in a specific package and to experience it in a certain way, and wasn't getting it—and truth be told still haven't gotten it—but it doesn't matter, because He loves me. It's what the Bible says. God *is love*. It's who He is. It's what He does.

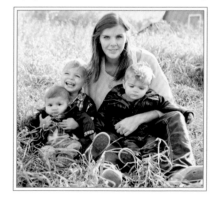

"I've come to realize that God loves me the way a parent loves their children. Like a child, I have thrown temper tantrums when I don't get what I want or what I expected and I think God looks at me in the same loving way, 'Oh Kristen, if only you knew how I am helping you, and teaching you, and growing you.'"

God's love is the perfect Christmas gift.

The Perfect Gift

Close your eyes
And I will sing a song for you.
I will always be there,
I will always love you.
And while you're dreaming
I will row your boat ashore.
I will always be there for you
Across the sky and back again.
We get torn and who knows when
My heart had begun to melt
All because of you.
I still fall apart
When you are in my arms like this.
You gave me the perfect gift.

Don't be scared to face your fears,

Don't be scared to spread your wings,

Don't be scared to share your tears,

'Cause love is everything.

And when you're dancing

you will never dance alone.

I will always be there.

If you remember all of this

You'll give me the perfect gift.

You gave me the perfect gift.

(John Cameron)

REFLECTION

- God's kind of love is unconditional. You cannot earn it. It's not related to your performance. It is a gift, freely given to you. "*God so loved the world that He gave His one and only Son…*" (John 3:16) Change your practice: stop trying to do things to earn God's love.

- Maybe you have believed in God for a long time but like Kristen, you've never taken in the truths of the songs you sing. Spend some time with the words of *Jesus Loves Me* and reflect on God's love for you, just as you are.

Lord, I start by believing that you love me. I accept the gift of your love. Today, I choose to not only accept your love for me but to give your love away to others I encounter. Thank you. I love you.

CHAPTER 3

Snow-Covered Pinecones & Snowflakes

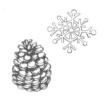

"This is the 'test' part of my testimony. I'm just trying to walk it out day by day, hand in hand, with a God who is so willing to guide me if I'll just say, 'I trust you. I believe.'" - Kristen

"No trial has overtaken you that is not faced by others. And God is faithful: He will not let you be tried beyond what you are able to bear, but with the trial will also provide a way out so that you may be able to endure it." 1 CORINTHIANS 10:13, NET

Mike and Kristen were married on September 25, 2004. Kristen walked down the aisle to the strains of the song "Come What May." Like all couples, they exchanged commitments to love "for better or for worse, in good times and bad, in sickness and in health." Little did they realize how significant those promises would be, and how much a man of his word Mike would need to be.

For Kristen, Christmas wasn't Christmas without snow. She introduced Mike to snow-covered pinecones and snowflakes as ornaments for their Christmas trees. But even for Kristen, the good thing about snow was that it's temporary. C.S. Lewis in his beloved book *The Lion, the Witch and the Wardrobe* imagined the most troubled country as a place where it was "always winter and never Christmas."

Trouble is temporary too. However, for Kristen and Mike, who had celebrated the birth of their first son, Beckett in 2008, things changed in 2009 and it seemed like the winter of their troubles had come to stay. Kristen called it the "test" part of her testimony.

> Trouble is temporary too. However, for Kristen and Mike, it seemed like the winter of their troubles had come to stay.

In March 2009, Mike's mother was diagnosed with kidney cancer. She passed away four short months later in July.

That same July, Kristen's sister-in-law Melanie, who happened to be the palliative care nurse for Kristen's mother-in-law, received news that her younger sister, Kaitlin, had a brain tumour. (After a brave battle, Kaitlin would pass away the following May at the age of seventeen, having changed the lives of many by using her "make a wish" to provide water wells for children in Uganda.)

In the fall of 2009, Kristen became pregnant with her second son, Tayven. He was born June 4, 2010. Then, in August 2010 Kristen was diagnosed with kidney cancer, thirteen months after her mother-in-law passed away from the same disease.

Kristen was scheduled to have surgery on the tumor in November 2010. Then life threw yet another curve ball: Kristen was pregnant with baby number three! When she saw the results of the pregnancy test, her stomach dropped. She didn't know what surgery plus pregnancy would look like, and she wasn't sure she wanted to find out. It sounded scary, and yet in the next instant she felt only peace, and in the corners of her heart had a sense that "This baby is going to be okay."

Kristen instantly phoned her doctor and was presented with a list of options:

a) She could wait to have surgery until after the baby was born, but then she would possibly miss her chance for a cure and die;

b) She could have surgery *while* she was pregnant. The potential existed that the painkillers and the anæsthetic would have an adverse effect on the baby and could leave her baby severely handicapped;

c) She could terminate the baby and proceed with cancer treatment.

What a heart-wrenching conversation.

Kristen said, "Here I am looking for advice and guidance from a professional and none of the options he has listed sound good to me at all. Thank goodness for other doctors in my life that I could call and talk to. I got off the phone with my doctor and went straight into the arms of Mike and cried, 'This is all too much!'"

Kristen and Mike decided to have the surgery while she was still five months pregnant. The surgery was performed on February 1, 2011 and everything went well. Eight weeks after her surgery she went to see her doctor so he could check her incision. He told her she had healed well and that the margins around where the tumour had been were clear. That was great news!

Kristen's third son, Lincoln, was born on June 13, 2011—at a whopping nine pounds, five ounces, he was a very healthy baby!

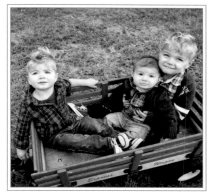

TAYVEN, LINCOLN AND BECKETT

After a person has had cancer, six-month post-operative checkups are routine. Kristen went for her first checkup in August 2011, fully expecting that they would tell her everything looked great and send her on her merry way.

That was not what happened.

Her ultrasound revealed that she had some very swollen lymph nodes around her kidney that looked suspicious. A further CT scan showed that the cancer was back and that it had spread to her lymph nodes, spine and left lung.

Kristen met with her surgeon. He sat her down and matter-of-factly told her the cancer was not operable. He informed her she had only one to two years left to live.

So how did Kristen face her troubles?

Kristen prayed.

She asked others to pray for her. Her name went out around the world to people who believe God answers prayer.

She asked for the leaders of her church to anoint her with oil and pray for her according to the instructions given in James 5:14.

She read and believed God's promises of healing from the Bible.

Kristen chose to follow the Gerson Therapy. This therapy activates the body's ability to heal itself through an organic, vegetarian diet, raw juices, coffee enemas and natural supplements. The Gerson Therapy treats the underlying causes of disease: toxicity and nutritional deficiency. Kristen essentially went on a ten-month fast. Mike and Kristen travelled to Mexico in February 2012 to spend fourteen days at a Gerson clinic.

She was supported by family and dear friends.

She trusted God.

Kristen's watchword in the winter of her soul became, "Lord, I trust you. I believe."

She said, "I do feel like I have the license to say, 'Wow, life hasn't been easy' and yet I *love* my life. I say that because God has literally been carrying me through, and He continues to hold me in the palm of His hand—and who wouldn't love that?"

> "I love my life. I say that because God has literally been carrying me through."

REFLECTION

- Are you facing the winter of your soul? Have troubles started piling onto your life? Does it appear that they are here to stay? Declare that whatever troubles you are facing have come into your life to pass. Claim a trust in God that is solid.
- Have you ever made promises that are hard to keep? How does your faith enable you to be a person of your word?

Lord, I feel like I am under a heavy load. There does not appear to be any end in sight to my problems. So, I make a choice today. I choose to believe that you are my provider. I believe that you are bigger than all my problems and my fears. I trust you. Lead me and protect me. Sustain me until these troubles have passed. Thank you.

CHAPTER 4

Orphan Ornaments

Mike and Kristen got matching tattoos
– "NEVER FORSAKEN"

"The LORD is compassionate and gracious, slow to anger, abounding in love." PSALM 103:8

"...Never will I leave you; never will I forsake you."
HEBREWS 13:5

Everyone has their own unique Christmas traditions. Kristen and Mike loved going to antique sales at Christmas time. Taking their time to leisurely meander around the displays was their way of finding calm in the craziness of the Christmas season. They always had their eyes out for Christmas ornaments, but not just any ornaments—they had to be ones that everyone else had passed over.

Their search was always an adventure because they were never quite sure what they were looking for—but they would know it when

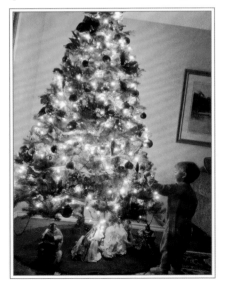

they saw it. One year it was a small glass ball with a snowman drawn on it with a dried out permanent marker, someone's unsuccessful attempt at creativity. The ornament sat forsaken on a shelf, until Kristen showed up—and then it found a home. Kristen and Mike affectionately dubbed their annual selections "orphan ornaments."

The journey of cancer can leave a person feeling like an unwanted ornament—marginalized, alone and forsaken. In such moments of isolation, Kristen found inspiration in the Bible.

Early on in her journey she was faced with making a decision on which course of treatment to follow. Kristen felt conflicted, not over the fear that she would make the choice that wouldn't save her life, but she wanted more than anything to make a choice that would honor God. She wanted to obey Him and so she prayed for wisdom. God quickly brought to her mind verses that settled her spirit.

> She wanted more than anything to make a choice that would honour God. She wanted to obey Him and so she prayed for wisdom.

"...*Never will I leave you; never will I forsake you*" (Hebrews 13:5).

"*The Lord is compassionate and gracious, slow to anger, abounding in love*" (Psalm 103:8).

Kristen said of these verses, "I closed my eyes, just pondering all the characteristics listed in the Psalm until they settled in my heart. As I lay there thinking, a picture or a scene came to my mind.

"I was a little girl, pigtails and all—say four-ish—and there I was, holding Jesus' hand, and we were walking on a *huge* Bible and He was just guiding me, pointing out things in His word, as if to say, 'Look what I did here…' and 'Kristen, look over here at what I did…' and we just walked all over that Bible as he showed me things.

"Then I saw another scene: Again, I was a little girl. Jesus was kneeling next to me with his hand around my waist. I stood next to him and then it was like he gave me a gentle little push, as if to say 'Go.' I took a few steps ahead and then stopped – as many children do when they are prompted to do something on their own. I stopped and looked back with hesitation. Jesus smiled and gave me a little 'go on' kind of look, but I didn't. I went running back to Him. I could see I was telling him all my worries and concerns and He just looked at me with that loving smile on his face as he patiently listened.

> "God's word has everything I need to know, and holds the power to accomplish it in my life. God knows all of my concerns with this whole decision, and listens patiently when I pour out my heart to him."

"As I opened my eyes and thought about these scenes, the first part struck me as a summary of the last nine months of my life. God has been taking me through His Word and teaching me and showing me His ways, and all the incredible things He did, and still does.

"The second part reminded me of my boys and me: I teach them the things they need to know, show them what needs to be done and the tools they will need to accomplish whatever it is. But I don't *do* it for them—I show them, and then let them go on their own.

"I also liked the knowing look on Jesus' face when 'Little Girl Kristen' was telling him her concerns. It's like when my boys come and tell me things that I already know. I look at them with a smile on my face, and give them my best 'Oh!? Really!? *Wow*!' not just to humor them.

"God's word has *everything* I need to know, and holds the power to accomplish it in my life. God *knows* all of my concerns with this whole decision, and listens patiently when I pour out my heart to him.

"I got up and got myself ready for bed, still thinking these things over, and feeling a sense of peace and relief. God isn't going to get mad at me, just like I don't get mad at my boys when they make a choice.

"As I crawled into bed that night, God brought my tattoo to mind *[After Kristen's cancer diagnosis, she and Mike had* gotten matching tattoos on their side, the words 'Never Forsaken'.] God was like, 'Kristen, what does your side say?'

"'Never Forsaken,' I replied in my heart.

"Right. 'Never will I leave you; never will I forsake you.'

"Then I heard Him say, 'What does *my* side say?'

"As I lay there thinking about it, my eyes welled up with tears. I thought of the verse that said, '*But he was pierced for our transgressions, he was crushed for our iniquities; the punishment that brought us peace was on him, and by his wounds we are healed* (Isaiah 53:5).

"Never forsaken."

REFLECTION

- Do you feel isolated or alone in your circumstances? Do you feel like no one else really understands what you are going through? Have you felt like you are failing? Ask God to bring to your mind a picture of his personal provision for you.

- Ask God to help you be aware of others in need in your own family or people who are close to you. How does God want you respond to the needs around you?

Lord, you have my attention. I need you. I claim your provision for me. Thank you that you are leading me. You are with me. You will never leave me or forsake. Thank you.

CHAPTER 5

Christmas Lights

The next step is to trust.

"...let your light shine before others, that they may
see your good deeds and glorify your Father in
heaven." MATTHEW 5:16

"Now faith is confidence in what we
hope for and assurance about what we do not see."
HEBREWS 11:1

Lights were essential ornaments on the Miller and Fersovitch family Christmas trees. Earlier Christmases saw multi-colored lights as the preferred choice but over the past few years, Kristen favored clear or white lights. However, one aspect that was consistent throughout the years was that there would *never* be any blinking lights on Kristen's tree.

Kristen firmly believed that a Christmas tree is supposed to be soothing. It is a work of art that could simply be appreciated in se-

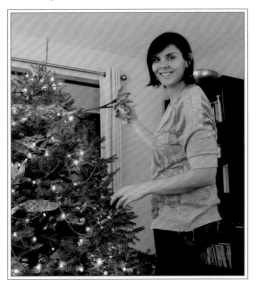

renity. Lights that flashed off and on were too busy for her. Only on The Singing Christmas Tree could she tolerate the "light show" and that was only because the Tree wasn't in Kristen's living room. Maybe you can relate.

Christmas is a season of welcoming the light. Even the Jewish celebration of Hanukkah around the time of the Christmas season is a "Festival of Lights." Light is good. Evil is usually associated with darkness. Light exposes what the darkness composes.

Revelation is also associated with light. New ideas are illustrated by a light bulb coming on. Inspiration is sometimes referred to as "illumination." Obeying truth is described as "walking in the light."

The development of faith "lightens" a person's life in more ways than one. Faith lessens the weight of life's loads. Faith also opens our eyes to trust.

Kristen had had faith in God since she was a child. Her parents prayed with her at mealtimes and bedtimes. They went to church together. They read their Bible together. Kristen's experiences in Sunday School, Youth Group, and on a Youth With a Mission Team trip in her young adult years all contributed to building her faith. Yet, it was the onset of cancer that drove her faith to a deeper level in God. Suffering has a way of doing that.

During her cancer journey, she had close encounters with God. One such encounter occurred as she prepared for her performance in the 2011 Singing Christmas Tree. I'll let her tell the story in her own words:

"This afternoon I was downtown at City Centre Mall picking up part of my outfit for The Singing Christmas Tree. It was lunch hour so everyone from the offices was out, and it was a madhouse. I couldn't get over how loud it was with music playing and everyone talking and laughing. It was *so* busy. Everyone seemed to be on a mission.

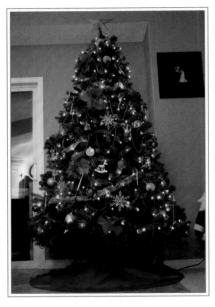

As I walked through the crowd, watching hundreds of people walk past me, I couldn't help but think, 'You never know what people are going through.'

"Through the buzz of everyone talking it was literally impossible to make out any conversation and yet it happened.

"A group of three ladies were heading towards me, with one of them talking to the other two. As these ladies got about five feet away from me, it was like I tapped into their conversation and couldn't

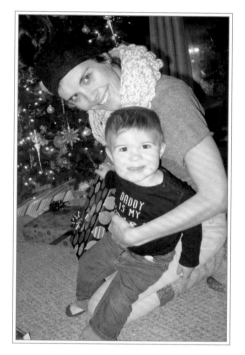

hear anything else, even though the craziness of the mall was still around, and I heard this lady say, 'The next step is to trust.'

"And that was it. That was all I heard. It happened in a matter of seconds and yet it seemed like it was slow motion. She said it, I heard it, and we walked in our opposite directions. She never knew the impact of her words.

"In that moment, I knew those words were for me: the next step is to trust.

"As I walked away a smile crossed on my lips, and I couldn't help but think and be reminded that trusting God isn't just a one-day decision and then it's 'easy peasy' from there. It's *every day*. The ups and downs, good and bad. Trust is a choice in every moment and every circumstance. Sometimes it's easy to trust, other times it's not at all.

"Trust is all He is asking from us and He'll take care of the rest. It's a choice. Faith doesn't always match what your head is telling you, but it is something you *know* in your heart."

Kristen felt these words from the Bible fit her circumstances perfectly:

> *"We were under great pressure, far beyond our ability to endure, so that we despaired of life itself. Indeed, we felt we had received the sentence of death. But this happened that we might not rely on ourselves but on God, who raises the dead. He has delivered us from such a deadly peril, and he will deliver us again. On him we have set our hope that he will continue to deliver us, as you help us by your prayers. Then many will give thanks on our behalf for the gracious favor granted us in answer to the prayers of many."*
>
> —2 CORINTHIANS 1: 8–11

REFLECTION

- Are you feeling under great pressure? Do you have faith in God but feel like it may not be sufficient to get you through? What is God saying to you about trusting Him in these circumstances?

- Have you ever been aware of times God has spoken to you, even in unusual circumstances? How have you responded?

Lord I believe what you say. You say that some things happen in my life so that I can rely on you. I like my independence but I have a greater need to depend on you. If you can raise the dead, and I believe you can, then you will see me through today. You will give me success and strength and in addition, make me a blessing to those around me. Thank you.

CHAPTER 6

Poinsettias

Poinsettias are known as the "Christmas Star." The star-shaped leaf pattern is said to symbolize the Star of Bethlehem.

"Magi from the east came to Jerusalem and asked, 'Where is the one who has been born king of the Jews? We saw his star when it rose and have come to worship him'…and the star they had seen when it rose went ahead of them until it stopped over the place where the child was. When they saw the star, they were overjoyed." MATTHEW 2:1,2, 9,10

Kristen and her mom decorated their Christmas trees with red and golden poinsettias. The yellow flowers at the centre of poinsettias are surrounded by brilliant red bracts, or modified leaves, and resemble large stars. That's why poinsettias are known as the "Christmas Star."

The star of Bethlehem led the magi many miles across the desert on their journey in search of a newborn king. It was no coincidence that the star appeared the way it did. It caught their attention and they embarked on a journey into the unknown. Then, just as they neared their destination, it disappeared only to appear again at just the right time. They were "overjoyed." No coincidence; it was God's providence—His timely care. God works in sovereign ways to arrange circumstances for our good.

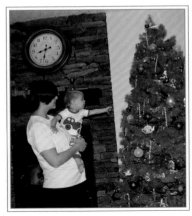

On June 6, 2013, Kristen texted me, "I'm just en route to the Cross [cancer hospital]. Guess what?? The EMS guy who is transferring me goes to North Pointe! And totally

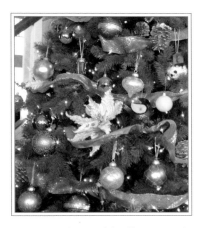

knows me and was so happy to be helping me and taking me! *Godwink!*"

"Godwink" had become a part of our church's vocabulary after Kristen introduced me to a book entitled *Divine Alignment*. Its author, Squire Rushnell, coined the term "Godwink" to describe what some people would call a coincidence, an answered prayer or simply an experience where you'd say, "Wow, what are the odds of that!" Godwinks are a way of seeing coincidences not as random acts that get our attention for a moment, but as intentional reminders from the Lord that He is at work, daily directing our lives.

Kristen had a Godwink in finding the *Divine Alignment* book. A friend had suggested she would love it. A few days later, while Kristen was waiting for an appointment, she happened to go into a store to pass the time. She noticed a bookrack and as she perused the selections, she saw a book on the bottom rack. It was *Divine Alignment*. "Hey, I heard about that book!" she thought and purchased it. She read one chapter and called me to ask if I had heard of it.

When I said no, she replied, "Well, Pastor Bob, you should get it." I did and it opened up a whole new perspective on life's coincidences.

Godwinks have a supernatural quality. They serve as guidance, warning, affirmation or creative inspiration. In times of *uncertainty* when what we desire more than anything else is *certainty*, Godwinks have a way of shoring up certainty.

The "EMS guy" Kristen mentioned was Ken Simmonds who had started to attend North Pointe in the fall of 2011. He and his family had been unsuccessfully looking for an Edmonton area church they could enjoy attending. His wife Rebecca's first Sunday at North Pointe happened to be the day Kristen shared her diagnosis of cancer and then sang a duet with Cindy Keating, the song "Unredeemed." Rebecca said that after hearing Kristen, she thought to herself, "If she is the kind of person that attends this church, then I want to attend here too!" That was a Godwink for Rebecca.

> Godwinks have a supernatural quality. They serve as guidance, warning, affirmation, or creative inspiration.

Ken's Godwink would come June 6, 2013 when he received a request to transport a "Fersovitch, K. age 29" to the Cross Cancer Hospital. He wondered if it might be "our Kristen." Sure enough, when he arrived, he saw Kristen waiting for her ride. "Hi," he said. "My name is Ken. Are you Kristen? Don't you go to North Pointe?"

When she said yes, Ken hugged her. Now, that is not his usual behaviour with patients but he was *so* happy to be helping her that he couldn't help himself.

His EMS partner was delayed so it gave Ken and Kristen time to talk about her family, about her husband Mike being a firefighter, her faith and North Pointe. When it came time to go, she picked up her purple pillow and off they went to the Cross Cancer Hospital.

On the way to the hospital, a song came on the radio. It was one that Kristen liked so she started to sing along—and Ken joined her, much to the surprise of his partner! Ken remembers Kristen as "the kind of person that when you enter her room you feel immediately at ease with her. She was such a positive and happy patient. That doesn't happen a lot. She was always smiling."

Kristen often encountered people in public who had previously connected with her in some way. Those moments were always uplifting for her and created the certainty of God's oversight of her life. She had no idea how many thousands of people her life touched, but God had a way of giving her glimpses. She said, "It's so funny how God works, and plans the people you are to meet within a day."

At one medical appointment Kristen had to get a CT scan. The nurse doing her IV recognized Kristen from a local newspaper article.

Another Godwink occurred on May 17, 2013 when Kristen had surgery. The nurse assisting the doctor recognized Kristen from The Singing Christmas Tree. She had been touched by Kristen's song and was so happy to help Kristen. So during the procedure they talked about The Tree, music and faith.

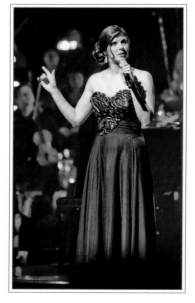

One Sunday when Kristen was feeling low, she met a pregnant woman in the foyer of North Pointe. The expectant mom told Kristen that if her baby was a girl she was going to name her Kristen because she wanted her daughter to grow up to have the same kind of strength that Kristen had. Kristen felt encouraged and humbled at the same time—and she got to meet her namesake, baby Kristen a few months later.

Godwinks assure us that:

- *I am part of a universe that is ordered and designed;*

- *My life is not an accident;*

- *There is a bigger picture than what I can see;*

- *Nothing happens by pure chance or accident, and what appears to be merely a fortunate or unfortunate circumstance is really the outworking of God's plans;*

- *Nothing enters my life that has not first passed through the hands of my loving heavenly Father.*

Those statements take into account the accidents, tragedies and disasters that violently rip away the lives of people we cherish. God is in the good and the terrible. In trying to sift our way through the wreckage left by loss, there is solace in knowing that life may be unfair but not out of control. Strength comes from realizing that there is more to life than meets the eye. None of us are guaranteed a long life or a pain-free one. We are guaranteed an eternal life by trusting in Jesus' sacrificial death and His resurrection.

> There is a bigger picture than what I can see.

Believing that God is sovereign does not mean everything will turn out well for us or lessen the pain of loss. It does mean that trusting God makes sense regardless of how things turn out.

"If you don't know what you're doing, pray to the Father. He loves to help. You'll get his help, and won't be condescended to when you ask for it. Ask boldly, believingly, without a second thought. People who 'worry their prayers' are like wind-whipped waves"

—JAMES 1:5–6, MSG

REFLECTION

- Have you attributed the "what-are-the-odds-of-that" moments in your life to coincidence? How do you see things differently if you think of such circumstances as providing evidence that God is in control?

- Look back over the course of the past forty-eight hours and take note of events or circumstances that may have seemed random but were intended to get your attention.

Lord, show me the fingerprints of your work on my life. I want to become more aware of what you are doing on my behalf. I ask for your wisdom and insight. I believe you will show me your ways. Thank you.

CHAPTER 7

A Wooden Rocking Horse

"Regardless of how bad things get, you can still be a joyous person, and I know that personally."

"Consider it pure joy, my brothers and sisters, whenever you face trials of many kinds, because you know that the testing of your faith develops perseverance." JAMES 1:2,3

Kristen had more ornaments than she could find room for on her tree. Even Beckett's lamb made its way onto their Christmas tree one year. Some ornaments made their way onto or off the tree each year, depending on how she felt. However, there were some non-negotiable ones. She had purchased ornaments for every special occasion in her and Mike's lives. There was the one celebrating their first year of marriage. A baby ornament was added when her son Beckett was born. Two more joined the first one with the arrivals of her younger boys, Tayven and Lincoln.

One other ornament had sentimental value, not because it commemorated anything special but because of its unique resil-

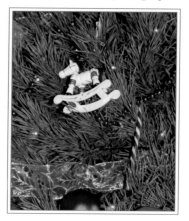

iency. It was a white, wooden rocking horse. Kristen would put it on her tree each year, and invariably sometime during the Christmas season it would get knocked off and break. Year after year the pattern was repeated. The horse was glued back together "a million times" according to Mike's calculations.

The resiliency of the rocking horse matched Kristen's own. She endured more adversity in her life than some people face in a hundred years. Her resilience is what endeared her to those who knew her best.

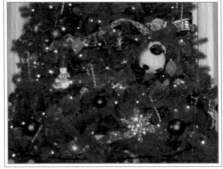

BECKETT'S LAMB

Kristen was a champion. The secret of every champion, whether in business, sport, love, finance or relationships is this ability to bounce back from setbacks. Champions have the same problems others do, but they get back up while others stay down.

The secret to Kristen's resilience was joy. When Elizabeth Withey interviewed Kristen in December 2011 for *The Edmonton Journal*, she was impressed by Kristen's attitude: "Kristen Fersovitch has endured more hard times in the past four years than many people see in a lifetime, yet she remains unflappably happy." Kristen had made a commitment to sing at a Prayer Rally in June 2013 but she was hospitalized for treatment at that time. Undaunted, Kristen got a day pass and along with her mom and Kennedy sang the Lord's Prayer at the rally. Many of the 700 people in attendance said they had never heard the Lord's Prayer sung so majestically and joyfully. That was the Spirit of God at work through Kristen.

Joy is not happiness. Joy actually creates happiness. Joy is spiritual, not just emotional. It's an attitude and an action. Feelings always follow actions. You can act your way into happiness faster than feel your way into happiness. The Bible often tells us to rejoice in God. To rejoice is a choice. Rejoicing is looking for God's influence in every situation of life and pointing out that influence to others. Rejoicing in the Lord is a change in perspective and outlook. Kristen's joy came from deep within her spirit. Her joy originated in her choice to trust and obey God, "*He* is the one that has brought me the joy that I get to sing about."

Kristen learned a Bible verse as a teen that served her well all of her life. "*...keeping our eyes fixed on Jesus, the pioneer and perfecter of faith. For the joy set out for him he endured the cross...*" (Hebrews 12:2). She could relate to Jesus. She drew strength from the same joy He focused on. She understood that her faith was being

> Rejoicing is looking for God's influence in every situation of life and pointing out that influence to others.

perfected by Jesus. This "perfecting" was a stretching process and not without its own kind of pain. She faced doubts and frustrations. At times, there seemed to be more frustrations than celebrations for her.

"There have been times when I've bawled my face off at the thought of my sons not having me. But regardless of how bad things get, you can still be a joyous person, and

> "Regardless of how bad things get, you can still be a joyous person, and I know that personally. I think that's something anyone can have."

I know that personally. I think that's something anyone can have."

Kristen felt frustrated more than fearful—frustrated because the only changes in her health were bad ones. Yet even in those times she would dig down deep and look up. "But I'm here. Maybe not doing the things I usually would, but I can count blessings abundant even in the place I'm at, and for that I am beyond grateful."

At one point Kristen was voicing her concerns and opinions to the Lord. "I was going on and on, and finally at the end of my prayer I remember saying, 'Well… clearly you know more than I do, and I don't understand, but I trust you. Your ways and thoughts are higher than mine… just speak to me Father, bring me comfort."

She grabbed her Bible and opened it up to Isaiah:

"For my thoughts are not your thoughts, neither are your ways my ways," declares the Lord. "As the heavens are higher than the earth, so are my ways higher than your ways and my thoughts than your thoughts… You will go out in joy

ORNAMENT

and be led forth in peace; the mountains and hills will burst into song before you, and all the trees of the field will clap their hands."

—ISAIAH 55:8, 9, 12

REFLECTION

- How can you experience joy? Are you looking for God's influence in every area of your life? Do you consistently look for reasons to thank or praise God, even when your own circumstances are difficult to endure?

- Do you ever feel like the broken rocking horse ornament? How has God helped you rise from your falls? How has He mended you?

Lord, open my eyes to see your influence in my life today. In this moment I thank and praise you for who you are. I believe that your ways are best and that you have my best interests in your heart. I trust you. Thank you.

CHAPTER 8

Candy Canes &
Lindor™ Chocolates

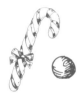

"I lost my life long ago. I gave it to Jesus."

"...*Whoever loses their life for me will find it.*"
MATTHEW 16:25

Why Lindor™ chocolates as ornaments? Kristen loved chocolate. (What woman doesn't?) Mike loved chocolate. (What firefighter doesn't?) Those were reasons enough.

Why candy canes as ornaments? The candy cane has become almost as much a part of Christmas as snow. In fact the candy cane was "invented" because of Christmas, but that's a story for another time.

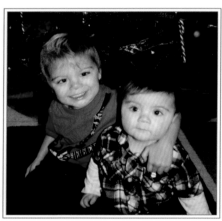

BECKETT AND TAYVEN

"Why?" is a good question. It's a question that helps define purpose. Knowing your purpose and living it out keeps you on track for a life of significance.

Why is also the title of a book. The *Why* book was produced for the people of Edmonton in 2013 and included Kristen's story, along with those of sports heroes, business professionals and politicians. It's a book that helps people find answers to questions like "Why am I here on Earth?" or

"Why is there so much suffering?" or "If there is a God and He is good, why do so many bad things happen?" The *Why* book began to be distributed on October 10, 2013—the day of Kristen's funeral. Over 100,000 homes would receive a book in which Kristen talked about *life* on the day of her funeral. What are the odds of that?

It's too easy to conclude that Kristen's death was a defeat. People might say,

"She lost her life." "Her family lost her." "We lost her."

But Kristen would say, "I lost my life long ago. I gave it to Jesus." She believed she had actually found her life when she became a Christian, a follower of Jesus. She also found her purpose, although she did not completely realize it until later.

Kristen said, "At the beginning of 2013, my pastor challenged our congregation to come up with a word for the year 2013. This word would be something to hold onto throughout the year as a source of encouragement and to challenge personal growth. I thought that sounded like a great idea so, as Mike and I drove home from church that afternoon, I asked God the quick question: 'Lord, what is my word for 2013?'

"Nothing came to my mind or heart immediately so I left it at that. As the days went on and I thought about it more and more, I found the word that was constantly popping up in my mind was

"Purposeful." That sounded like a good word to me and even though I knew I had a fairly good idea of what the definition was, I figured I should look it up in the dictionary just in case there was something I was missing.

"It said:

pur·pose·ful (adjective)
1. having a purpose.
2. determined; resolute.
3. full of meaning; significant.[1]

"When I first read, 'having a purpose' I couldn't help but roll my eyes and think:

'Thank you, *Captain Obvious!*' I was slightly irritated by the fact that having a purpose was exactly what I have been trying to do, and I thought, "How can you be purposeful if you don't know what your purpose is!!!?

"You know those people you meet or see who are *exactly* where they need to be, and doing *exactly* what they should be doing, because they are *so* incredible at it? I have this desire to be like such a person, and yet realize that maybe not everyone can or is supposed to

---

1 "Purposeful". The Free Dictionary. June 6, 2015. (http://www.thefreedictionary.com/purposeful)

have that. Maybe some people are called to be good at a whole bunch of little things.

"Anyone who knows me, knows that I am a *dreamer!* When I was initially given the word 'purposeful' I instantly thought, *'Change the world!'* which was quickly followed by, '… but how??'

"As I mulled this over, I concluded that even if I didn't have or know my exact *purpose*, *but* that I would just try to be purposeful in all that I do. I would be determined, and try to have things be significant. I also threw in my own little definitions of 'moving forward,' 'putting in a conscious effort,' and 'living with intention.' So, with

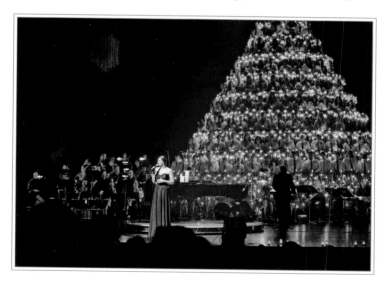

my new word in my heart and mind, I tried to put it into action for the simple everyday things in my life.

"One morning, Mike and I decided to take the boys and visit my sister Kennedy and her class at the school she works in. I thought it would be fun to bring her a coffee, and some flowers, and Kennedy knew her kids would just love visiting with the boys. Just as Kennedy expected, her grade threes loved the boys, and being the amazing teacher she is, Kennedy quickly incorporated the boys into the lesson with story time. When the story was finished, Kennedy asked the kids to guess what Mike did for a living – and after a few guesses of 'teacher,' 'dad,' 'farmer'... someone finally guessed 'firefighter.' This opened the opportunity for the kids to ask Mike all kinds of questions regarding his job.

"As I sat at Kennedy's desk in the corner of the room just watching and listening to these kids excitedly ask Mike questions, I was overwhelmed by the idea that Mike sharing his love for his job and the excitement and dangers that are involved with firefighting *could* be shaping one of these kid's lives.

"Of course we may never know for sure, but as we drove home I told my thoughts with Mike. I said, 'What seemed to be like a fun little visit to Kennedy's class room to bring her coffee and flowers, could have turned into *you* shaping the future of one of those kids... without even knowing it.'

"I could just imagine a grown up girl or boy from that class years down the road saying: 'In grade three this man came into my class, and his job as a firefighter sounded exciting, and from then on I knew that's what I wanted to be.'

"Mike didn't have his uniform on, or any of his gear. He looked like an ordinary guy wearing his jeans and a t-shirt, drinking a coffee, but to one of those kids, Mike could have been the ember (no pun intended) needed to inspire them to become a firefighter. All because in his ordinary day he took the *time* to answer their questions.

"In an ordinary day, by words of kindness and gentleness, or acts of love, graciousness and compassion, the encounters *you* have with people (friends, loved ones, or the cashier at the grocery store) could be the ember of hope *they* need to flame into their future or... they may be, an ember of hope, for you."

> "By words of kindness and gentleness, or acts of love, graciousness and compassion, the encounters *you* have with people ... could be the ember of hope *they* need to flame into their future."

The purpose of the candy cane? It's sweet and tastes good. There is no historical record that candy canes were created to communicate religious meaning, but it doesn't take much to draw the following illustrations from the candy cane:

- *The white colour symbolizes the sinless nature of Jesus.*

- *The candy's hardness symbolizes the firmness of the promises of God.*

- *The candy cane is formed as a "J" to represent the name of Jesus.*

- *The "J" also represents the staff of a "Good Shepherd."*

- *The red stripes show the stripes of the scourging Jesus received and his blood that was shed for our forgiveness.*

REFLECTION

- Who does God want me to influence? What opportunities may I be inclined to miss because I doubt my life matters to God?
- What is a word for the coming year that would help keep you focused and on track to achieve God's purposes for your life?

Lord, I believe, help my unbelief. Today, I choose to believe that my life matters. You created me for a purpose. I want to make my life count. Thank you.

CHAPTER 9

Red Beads &
Golden Ribbon

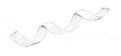

"Hope is not the conviction that something will turn
out well, but the certainty that something makes
sense, regardless of how it turns out."
VACLAV HAVEL

"...we know that suffering produces perseverance;
perseverance, character; and character, hope. And
hope does not put us to shame..." ROMANS 5:3-5

Kristen would drape her Christmas trees with garlands of red beads and golden ribbon. Garlands have been used around the world and in most cultures to celebrate festive occasions. Often the first garland formed by children is a daisy chain and Kristen made a few in her day. She loved the garlands on her own trees.

The Bible compares the instruction and teaching of parents to a garland. "*They are a garland to grace your head…*" (Proverbs 1:9). The proverb teaches that when children listen and obey the good instructions of their parents out of respect, it's a beautiful thing like a garland.

Sometimes Kristen found this challenging. She had a strong stubborn streak to her. Actually it was more like a swath than a streak. The Miller home had some times of tension during Kristen's teen years, but that's true for many homes. Despite her challenges, Kristen respected her parents. Their values and beliefs helped shape the woman she became. Underlying all they taught her was a Christian worldview.

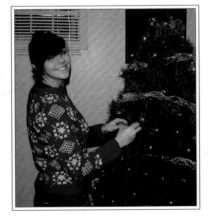

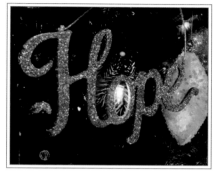

ORNAMENT ON MIKE'S DAD'S TREE

A large part of that worldview was rooted in hope—hope that there is more to life than meets the eye. It is a hope that says as tangible as our temporal world is, there is an even more real eternal realm. It is a hope that says, "Life is unfair but God is good." Life may not make sense at times, but it is temporary, and there is a grander purpose than just making it through life feeling comfortable. That's why sickness and a terminal prognosis couldn't defeat Kristen. She had hope.

In February 2013 Kristen was expressing her frustrations and feelings to a friend. During their conversation her friend asked, "How is your spirit feeling??" Kristen's response? "Hopeful. Somehow, always hopeful."

She recalled that conversation later and reflected, "The hope I feel reminds me of the wood-burning fireplace Mike and I have in our home. At night, before we go to bed, Mike will load that thing up and it will burn all night long, and in the morning the fire is out. You look inside and all you see is a heap of ashes. Spiritually I felt at times like that heap of ashes. Frustration, anger, fear, worry and the hardships of the journey had burned me out.

"One morning, after the fire had gone out, I decided I wanted another fire so I began to stir the ashes and dig

"Hopeful. Somehow, always hopeful."

a little bit, and there, in the very middle, was a tiny ember. Hope. I quickly recalled that conversation: 'somehow, always hopeful.'

"That morning I started a whole new fire with that little ember and was reminded it only takes a tiny ember to start a blazing fire."

"There was a peace she had that's hard to even understand," said Kristen's sister Kennedy Miller. "That has entirely to do with her faith and just trusting in God. She definitely found hope in her faith."

That's the beauty of hope. Vaclav Havel, the last president of Czechoslovakia, famously said, "Hope is not the conviction that something will turn out well, but the certainty that something makes sense, regardless of how it turns out."

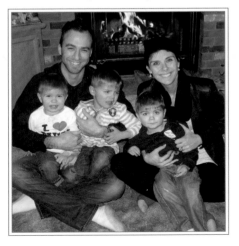

Hope meant that Kristen was prepared for death but at the same time wasn't ready to die. She was ready to live. Being prepared to face death did take away the fear of dying. She was certain that, if she was not healed and passed away, she would experience eternal life in heaven. The lyrics of her last song, sung just hours before her passing were, "I will praise Him, I will praise Him, Praise the Lamb for sinners slain, Give Him glory all you people, for His blood can wash away each stain."

> "God is *big*.
> Bigger than
> anything that would
> try to overcome you,
> or your family."

Kristen believed, "God is *big*. Bigger than anything that would try to overcome you or your family. I have come to know God as a provider, sustainer, giver of joy, and peace and so much more… and I am currently on a journey that is leading me to know him as my healer.

"But let's say I didn't get healed—what if I died? Would that mean that He wasn't God? No, not at all. We all are going to die; we are not invincible; we are human; we all make mistakes; we all fall short. But there is a God of grace and mercy who made you so He could love you. He loved you so much that he sent his son Jesus to die for you. For me.

"My life is preserved by Jesus, because He died for me, because I accepted Him as my Lord and Savior. He is the giver of life—*eternal* life—so when my time here on Earth is done, I get to

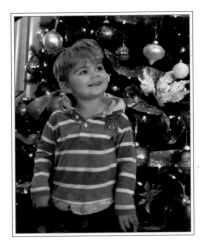

live in eternity with God. *That is what gets me through each day. That is what sustains, and brings peace and joy.*"

Just after her thirtieth birthday, Kristen breathed her last breath on Earth and breathed her first taste of heavenly air.

Imagine stepping onto a shore and finding it's Heaven.

Imagine taking hold of a hand and finding it's God's hand.

Imagine breathing new air and finding it's celestial.

Imagine feeling invigorated and finding its immortality.

Imagine passing from storms and tempest to an unknown calm.

Imagine waking up and finding it's home.

"I lift up my eyes to the mountains—where does my help come from? My help comes from the Lord, the Maker of heaven and earth. He will not let your foot slip – he who watches over you will not slumber; indeed, he who watches over Israel will neither slumber nor sleep. The Lord watches over you – the Lord is your shade at your right hand; the sun will not harm you by

day, nor the moon by night. The Lord will keep you from all harm – he will watch over your life; the Lord will watch over your coming and going both now and forevermore."

—PSALM 121

REFLECTION

- Do you feel hopeful? Do you believe that God is bigger than anything that can come against your life or your family? Do you have hope even the size of a small ember? How can you turn that ember into a fire of hope?
- No one is fully prepared to live until they are prepared to die. Are you prepared?

Lord, I want your hope in my life. Life is precious and I am not ready to die for a long time but I want to be prepared for death when it does come. So, help me live today to its fullest. Help me to glorify you in all I think and say and do. Thank you.

CHAPTER 10

A Gold Star

"My life is His, lived for His Glory, for His name...
because HE is the one that has brought me
the joy that I get to sing about." - Kristen

*"Well done, good and faithful servant! You have
been faithful with a few things; I will put you
in charge of many things. Come and share your
master's happiness!"* MATTHEW 25:23

Kristen's Christmas tree was crowned with a gold star. It was always the last ornament to go on the tree. The star reminded her of the star of Bethlehem. It also brought back memories of the gold stars

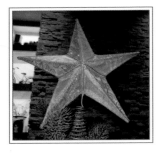

her elementary teachers would put on her schoolwork. She loved getting gold stars! They were recognitions of her achievement and she was proud of them.

In February 2013, Kristen received a "gold star" of a different sort. She found herself sitting with twenty-eight fellow Edmontonians who would receive the Queen's Diamond Jubilee Medal. As she listened to each of the biographies being read, she couldn't help but be moved by the people who surrounded her, the *incredible* things they had done for their communities, and how well they represented Canadians.

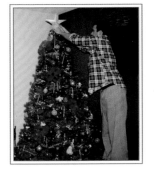

Among the other recipients was Reverend Mike Love who had been Kristen's youth pastor at Central Tabernacle. He was honored for his recent work with youth all over the world and the hundreds of thousands of youth and young adults he brings together annually for an annual youth convention to discover their God-given dreams. Another recipient was a woman who had served the Girl Scouts for more than thirty years, and another was a man who was recognized for his breakthrough research in autism.

> A brief life doesn't have to be an incomplete life.

"I'd be lying if I said I couldn't help but think, 'Man, I feel kind of puny around these people,'" Kristen said, as usual underestimating the impact she had made on people. She humbly received the medal from the hands of Mike Lake, Minister of Parliament for Edmonton Mill-woods-Beaumont along with his words of commendation.

Kristen's medal would later adorn a table of remembrance at her funeral. On October 10, Millwoods Assembly was filled with Kristen's family, friends, admirers and people touched by her story who had come to pay their respects and grieve together. The platform background consisted of black curtains covered in white pin lights. The effect looked like a wondrous starry night. Throughout the building were posters displaying the phrase *"Your One and Only Life."* The posters were in support of the church's current sermon series but they were a timely fit for Kristen's funeral.

We only get one life. Even though everyone wants to live a long life, the duration is not as important as the donation. A brief life doesn't have to be an incomplete life. Kristen courageously chose to bring honor to Jesus in the midst of her suffering. In doing so, she touched a world that is impressed less with how we handle suc-

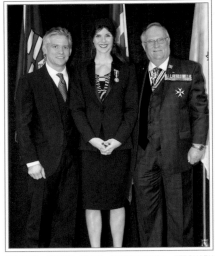

QUEEN'S JUBILEE MEDAL PRESENTATION, FEBRUARY 2013. THE HONOURABLE MIKE LAKE, MP, EDMONTON MILLWOODS-BEAUMONT, KRISTEN AND LIEUTENANT GOVERNOR OF ALBERTA DONALD S. ETHELL

cess than how we deal with suffering and adversity. Her one and only life shone brightly, if painfully.

Kristen told me there were times when she felt embarrassed or ashamed that she had not been healed of cancer. For her that meant that, in a world where people strive for perfection, it felt like she was failing. People prayed for healing and she was still sick. It must be her fault somehow. As ridiculous as that sounds, the condemning feelings were there.

> We may not be able to always trace God's hand in our lives but we can trust His heart. Kristen did.

Those are the lies of the enemy of our soul. If healing depended solely on the strength of a person's faith then Kristen would be still with us. If the quality of the people who pray, the quantity of their prayers and the amount of fasting and believing they did were what it took to move God's hand, then Kristen would be alive and well. Death doesn't mean we should give up on God. In fact, it should sober us to open our hearts to Him. We may not be able to always trace God's hand in our lives but we can trust His heart. Kristen did.

CTV News covered Kristen's funeral and noted a pair of women's running shoes prominently displayed on the platform. Kristen had kept those running shoes on her bedroom nightstand as a way of reinforcing the belief that she would use them again. In the spring of 2013 we talked about a day when she would be well enough to run. I promised I would run with her then and until then I would be praying for her every time I ran.

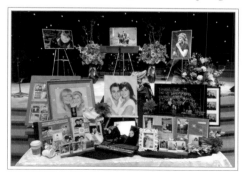

Although she didn't run in those shoes, Kristen ran her race.

She finished her course.

There is a crown laid up for her.

She ran a marathon of hope and crossed the finish line as a champion.

Her earthly accolades paled in comparison to the words, "Well done, Kristen, good and faithful servant," that she heard from Jesus.

There was a gold star not only the top of her Christmas tree but crowning her life. Well done, indeed.

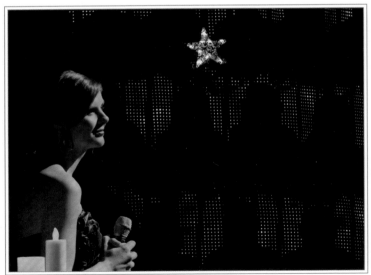

AFTER KRISTEN PASSED AWAY, THE DEC. 2013 TREE FEATURED THIS "PERMANENT" STAR, WHICH SHONE DURING EVERY PERFORMANCE IN MEMORY OF KRISTEN.

REFLECTION

- Who are you trying to please? Whose approval matters to you most? Are you conscious of your accountability to God? If you are fully aware of this, how will that awareness affect the choices you need to make today?

- Reflect on what it means to run the race well and consider God's approval for His good and faithful servants.

Lord, help me to live my life in the light of eternity. Remind me that I determine my destiny by the choices I make each day. Please give me your wisdom and the courage to do what you would have me do. Thank you.

CHAPTER 11

Christmas Without Kristen

The rest of the story…

"Where, O death, is your victory? Where, O death, is your sting?" 1 CORINTHIANS 15:55

The day after Kristen's funeral service, I had the privilege of accompanying her body south to Garth, Alberta with John Daviduck of Serenity Funeral Services. We made the two-hour drive through Mundare and past the world's largest mallard in Andrew. Garth Evangelical Cemetery is where Mike Fersovitch's mom was buried. We were the first on site. The sun was out and the wind wasn't too cold for early October. Kristen's extended family arrived from Bonnyville and Edmonton.

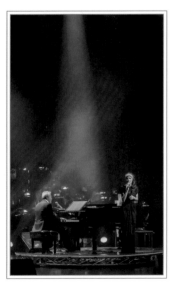

Kristen's favourite colour was green so Mike's cousin, Rebecca, had purchased three green, star-shaped balloons—one for each of Kristen's sons. They would release them in memory of their mom as their contribution to her service. A year earlier, Kristen had taken her own green balloon and released it as an act of hope, leaving her fears and worries about the future to God and watching the balloon float heavenward.

The time came in the service for each boy to release their balloon. What happened next was another Godwink. The wind caught the balloons and carried them towards a stand of trees by the cemetery. I wondered if their lift would get them high enough to clear the branches. As we all watched, the first two balloons cleared the treetops by inches and sped away. However, the third balloon got caught on a branch. There was an audible groan from those of us watching before we turned our attention back to the service.

> Where, O death, is your victory?

I was reading from the Bible in 1 Corinthians, chapter 15 about the defeat of death. As I read, I watched the balloon out of the corner of my eye. Just as I got to the phrase, *"Where, O death, is your victory?"* the wind came up and pried the last balloon free from the branch's grasp and it began to ascend. I excitedly said, "Look—it's free!" Everyone turned to see. I felt as though time stood still. The word "free" echoed in my mind. Kristen was free. She had left her earthly body behind. She finally knew what it was to be free. The cancer was gone. The pain was over. She was safe at home. She was more alive than she had ever been. Free indeed! I read the remaining verses through my tears.

Our prayers for Kristen's healing were not answered. Why? That's a legitimate question to ask. But if we knew the answer, would we like it? It wouldn't bring Kristen back. Would it help the grief any better than simply knowing that Kristen is in heaven? Like Kristen said, "He is the giver of eternal life so that when my time on earth is done I get to spend eternity with God."

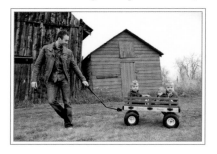

The better question is, "What?" What now? What will happen for Mike and the boys?

Mike says, "I have learned too well the value of life as of late, and try not to wish each day away so quickly so that time might ease the pain. My life is not full of depression and sadness. There are many moments of joy and laughter in our home, and when God joined Kristen and me together in marriage, He gave me more than death could ever take."

Mike adds, "The Bible says love is stronger than death.

Two thousand years ago God sent his Son to defeat death by dying ain our place.

There is no defeat in Kristen's death.

There is overwhelming grief and an ocean of tears.

"There are many moments of joy and laughter in our home, and when God joined Kristen and I together in marriage, He gave me more than death could ever take."

There is disappointment.

There are questions.

But there is no defeat."

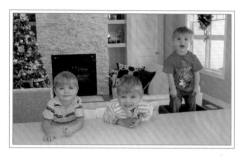

"My boys have been wonderful, and yes, they know Mommy is with Jesus. They are happy and as full of energy and curiosity as ever. We have been continually surrounded with family and friends and for that I am so very thankful. There are far too many people to thank who have been there for us and who continue to be there for my boys and me in this journey."

The Bible reveals the reality of heaven. Jesus said, "*I tell you, whoever hears my word and believes him who sent me has eternal life and… has crossed over from death to life*" (John 5:24).

REFLECTION

- Do you believe in heaven? Do you have hope that there is more to life than meets the eye?
- Love is stronger than death. Are there people in your life that need to know hear that from you?

Lord, I want to live freely today. Free to obey you and honour you in all I do. Bring the wind of your Spirit to bear on my circumstances and lift me up and set me free. Thank you.

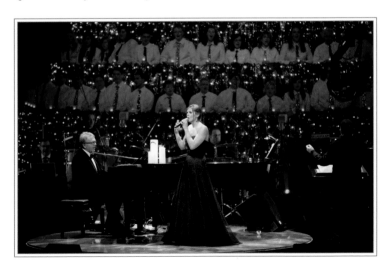

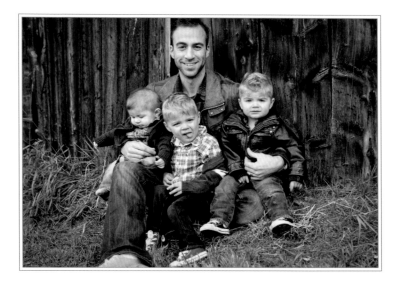

While this book is about Kristen, people wonder about the rest of the story with Mike and the boys. What will the rest of their story be? How will Mike use the principles he and Kristen followed in the marriage for his life without her?

These are Mike's personal thoughts:

"I can't imagine a fulfilling future that works without Kristen in it. That being said, I know that there is one in store for me—I just can't picture it yet. I can't quite see the light at the end of the tunnel, but I do know there is a light there. I have been given the strength to keep walking through this tunnel and there are many who walk with me: sometimes pushing, pulling or dragging me along.

"I have not come a long way forward without Kristen, but I have made some progress. This book talks about how Kristen and I pressed on through our journey of life. Even now these same principles continue to help me manage.

> When our faith seemed crushed, we would pray for more faith and remind ourselves that all we needed was a mustard seed-sized faith and we could move mountains.

"We leaned heavily on the Bible, the word of God. We would constantly remind ourselves and immerse ourselves in the healing power written about in the Bible. We would constantly encourage each other 'when one was weak the other was strong' (the words to one of Kristen's songs). When we felt broken and run down, Kristen would never be afraid to ask for help or prayer; she surrounded herself with prayer warriors. When our faith seemed crushed, we would pray for more faith and remind ourselves that all we needed was a mustard seed-sized faith and we could move mountains. Sometimes when the spiritual burden seemed too much to bear we would remember that no acts of our own or proper prayers or fasting could bring about healing: it is simply the grace of

God that is required to see her well. '*With man this is impossible, but with God all things are possible*' (Matthew 19:26).

"Kristen baffled the doctors so many times. A doctor would examine her scans before meeting her and then be in total amazement when she would come bouncing and smiling into an appointment. I once remember Kristen walking slowly toward a CT-scan machine and becoming aware of a multitude of medical staff standing behind a thick sheet of safety glass watching her. When she noticed them staring, she started this random silly little dance across the front of the glass on her way to the machine and had them all in hysterics.

"That all being said the end result was not what we hoped and prayed for. Kristen eventually succumbed to her illness and left so many of us with the question of, 'God why didn't you save her?' But is that the right question? I have since learned that the cancer Kristen had was a very rare form of kidney cancer. It is usually only found in children and in the most severe cases such as Kristen's, the child would die at a very early age. The strange thing is that Kristen was born with this already in her body and not only did she 'defy all odds' after her diagnosis, but she in all rights should have never even have survived past childhood. So maybe the question should not be, 'Why did she die?' but rather, 'Why did she live?' To me the answer is clear.

"The other day I went for a walk alone at sunset. As we live out in the country, I often enjoy the fresh air and beautiful skies. I was walking alone, basically in the middle of a farmer's field, when I spotted a lone truck slowly driving down an empty oil road several hundred meters adjacent to my path. This field is near my home and it's quite familiar to me. It's unusual to see a vehicle traveling so slowly at that time of the day. The thought occurred to me that this was not an oil field worker but most likely a hunter desperately seeking his last chances at having a success-

> So maybe the question should not be 'Why did she die?' but rather, 'Why did she live?'

ful hunt. I considered my own situation: brown coveralls, dark jacket with a fur-lined hood walking alone through an empty field at dusk. I began to become painfully aware of how desolate and possibly attractive I might look to an eager and overexcited hunter.

"My fears were greatly intensified as my awareness of this hunter seemingly coincided with his awareness of me. As our paths began to come closer together, my fears were realized when his truck slowed to a stop for no apparent reason. Unless, it was to examine me: his possible prey! My heart was beating fast and my imagination running wild. I could clearly picture the man pulling out his rifle and training his crosshairs on my body. I was nearly panic-stricken, wanting to lie down and hide or run to safety, but I know as a hunter that this would be typical for game to do as their animal instincts kick in when they sense danger.

"I decided in an attempt to save my life (at least in my own mind) to make myself look as human as possible. I waved my arms and stood tall, basically trying to look like a typical stick-man figure that anyone should recognize as human. In doing this, I also felt like I was making myself a bigger target and at any moment I expected everything to go black, or see my own blood on the snow.

"Thirty seconds went by, and then a minute, and I wasn't shot yet. I just felt too vulnerable (and silly) to stay any longer and so I decided to take my chances and turn my back and calmly walk away as the truck sat there staring at me with its lights out.

"As I started to walk, fear still gripped me, the same fears that often come out late at night when I miss Kristen and am left alone to wrestle with my thoughts. *What if something happens to me? What If I die? Who will watch the boys? What message would I want to leave my boys? How would I want their new parents to raise them?* Then it hit me. I could answer my own questions. I am still alive. I can tell my boys how much I love them any time I want! I can raise my children the way I would want someone else to raise them. We are quick to tell our babysitters to limit television time, sugar intake and fast food, etc. I want my children to be exposed often to prayer and the Bible. I want them to be taken diligently to church and encouraged in their faith in any way possible. I asked myself the question, 'Am I doing all of these things?' That was it! I had it! Plan A was to raise my kids the way I would want someone else to raise them. It is so ridiculously simple yet so incredibly tough to do at times. That is my first plan and that is how I will move forward.

> I could actually embrace and sense God's love and His plan for me and my boys' lives.

"During that same frightening walk as I began to approach my house and felt safe again, my mind began to replay what could have happened out in the field. I knew I was out of harm's way now and my thoughts seemed much clearer. I now felt that if I had been shot, at least it would most likely have been a quick death. I imagined myself going black and then waking up and lifting my head up from the ground at a bright beautiful sky and Kristen bending over me with a huge smile, saying, '*Hi!* I didn't expect to see you so soon!'

"As I continued to walk and my imagination continued to suspend me in paradise, I felt a sense of peace come into my heart. As Kristen and I stood there together in heaven, now in the full presence of the Lord, I had no fear for my boys left back on Earth. I knew God would be with them. I could actually embrace and sense God's love and His plan for me and my boys' lives. I felt assured that God not only dwells in heaven but He is also here with me on Earth. 'I will never leave you nor forsake you.' It was a great feeling!"

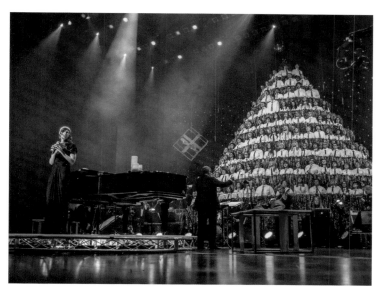

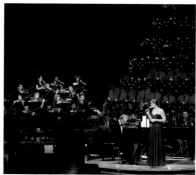

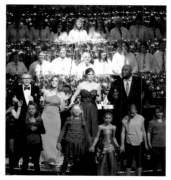

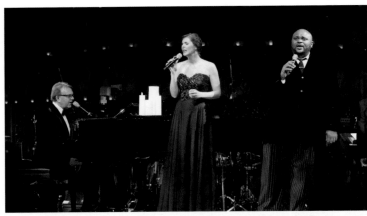

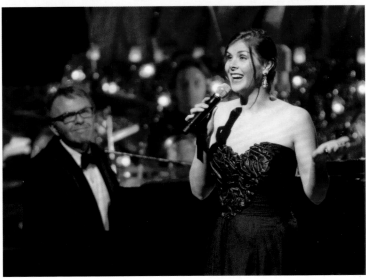

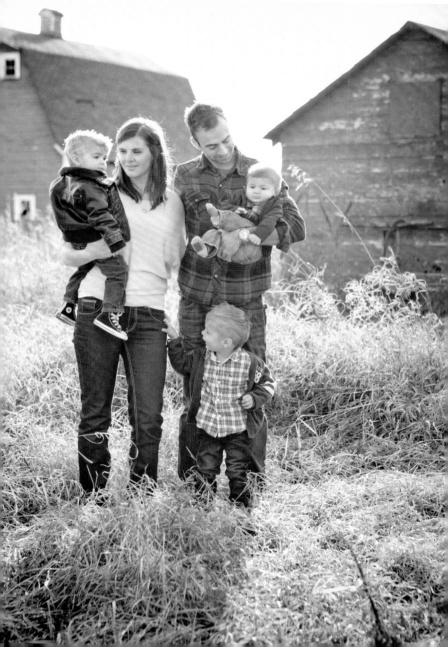

ORNAMENT

One of the meanings of the word "ornament" is: "A person considered as a source of pride, honour, or credit." Discovering that definition was an "aha" moment for me. Kristen perfectly fit that definition. She gave honor to what it is to be a Christian. My hope is that her story has motivated you to explore your own trust in God and keep an open mind to becoming a follower of Jesus.

REV. ROBERT W. JONES

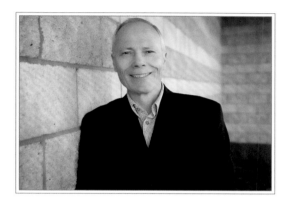

Rev. Robert W. Jones is the Senior Pastor of North Pointe Community Church (formerly Central Tabernacle). He helped produce eleven years of The Singing Christmas Tree and now serves on the Board of The Singing Christmas Tree Foundation.

North Pointe is the home church to Mike Fersovitch's family and Kristen's parents, Dave and Kathy Miller.

The Edmonton Singing Christmas Tree Foundation: I am forever grateful for the use of photos of Kristen in The Singing Christmas Tree, 2011, 2012 and for promoting this book at the 2013 Tree.

www.edmontonsingingchristmastree.com

John Cameron, Executive Producer of The Singing Christmas Tree: Thank you for your encouragement and support of this book. You inspire all of us with your generosity and dreams.

www.johncameron.com

Liz Boyer, Chalk: A friend of Kennedy Miller who generously donated her time to create the gorgeous images for each chapter and designed the covers and book. It was fantastic working with you!

www.studiochalk.ca

Kristy-Ann Swart, Up and Away Studios: Thank you for allowing the use of your photos of the Fersovitch family in this book. Your photography is superlative!

www.upandawaystudios.com

Katelyn Kimo, Production World: Thank you for compiling the photos of Kristen from The Singing Christmas Tree files.

www.productionworld.ca

Cindy Keating, Red Carpet Life: Thank you for inspiring the "Ornament" concept and your support behind the scenes in writing this book. Your love for Kristen endures.

www.cindykeating.com

Wendy Connors, Impact Orientations: Thank you for proof-reading the final version and for your helpful input.

www.impactorientations.com

Mike Fersovitch, Dave and Kathy Miller: Thank you for the coffee and memories that form the foundation of the content of this book. God bless and keep you as you raise Beckett, Tayven and Lincoln.